Essentia
Aromathe

Your Ultimate Guide to Getting Started and Safely Using Essential Oils to Beat Stress, Cure Your Ailments, Boost Your Mood and Provide Emotional Wellbeing

Essential Oils and Aromatherapy Basics
Your Ultimate Guide to Getting Started and Safely Using Essential Oils to Beat Stress, Cure Your Ailments, Boost Your Mood and Provide Emotional Wellbeing

By Sheila Mathison

Copyright © 2014 Softpress Publishing

Disclaimer:
The following statements have not been evaluated by the Food and Drug Administration. This product is not intended to diagnose, treat, cure, or prevent any disease. The advice and strategies contained herein may not be suitable for every situation. This work is sold with the understanding that the publisher is not engaged in rendering medical or other professional advice or services. The publisher does not specifically endorse any company or product mentioned or cited in this document. Websites listed were accurate at the time of publishing, but may have changed or disappeared between when it was written and when it is read.

No responsibility or liability is assumed by the publisher for any injury, damage or financial loss sustained to persons of property from the use of this information, personal or otherwise, either directly or indirectly. While every effort has been made to ensure reliability and accuracy of the information within, all liability, negligence or otherwise, from any use, misuse or abuse of the operation of any methods, strategies, instructions or ideas contained in the material herein, is sole responsibility of the reader.

All information is generalized, presented for informational purposes only and presented "as is" without warranty or guarantee of any kind.

All trademarks and brands referred to in this book are for illustrative purposes only, are the property of their respective owners and not affiliated with this publication in any way.

Table of Contents

Introduction

Essential oils provide us with a natural way to enhance our lives and heal our ailments. They have been used for thousands of years to cure our physical ailments, boost our moods and soothe our mental state. Essential oils were used long before modern medicines were even thought of and continue to be sought after to create relief from what ails us without all the undesirable and potentially harmful side effects contemporary pharmaceuticals can cause. These oils are beginning to make a comeback as more and more people seek out "organic" solutions to our body's disorders.

This book is intended to be an indispensable primer for anyone seeking to learn about Essential Oils from the most basic level. This beginner's guide contains a wealth of useful information gathered from reliable and highly regarded sources. Inside this comprehensive resource you will find numerous helpful tips and guidance on buying, storing, and using essential oils so you can get started on the right path with confidence. There is an entire chapter devoted to using essential oils on your body and another on uses for the oils around your home. I have even include a section outlining how to make your own oils to save a few dollars.

Also, don't miss my follow-up book, **Essential Oils and Aromatherapy Recipes: Natural Health and Beauty Solutions Using Essential Oils and Aromatherapy for Stress Reduction, Pain Relief, Skin Care, and Beauty**. I have carefully crafted this handy reference so you will receive maximum benefit in your daily life from the many advantages offered by essential oils. Inside this valuable resource you will find over **177 Recipes** for treating everything from sprains, to back pain, to headaches as well as useful, money-saving instructions for making your own toothpaste, lip balm, and hair care products, **plus tons more! Get it today!**

One last thing, as a way of saying Thank You for buying my book I have put together a **FREE GIFT** just for you!

i.

"28 Aromatherapy Recipes for Essential Oils"

This gift is the perfect complement to this book so just head over to this web address to get access.

http://www.softpresspublishing.com/aromatherapy

Chapter 1 - What Are Essential Oils?

Essential oils are the liquid derived from the aroma of various plants. In simple terms, they are the "oil of" the plant from which they were extracted. These oils are "essential" in the sense that they carry a distinctive scent, or essence, of the plant. The oils are typically extracted from the plant via distilling. Leaves, stems and flowers are typically used as the sources of the oil. However, some plants contain the desired properties in their roots and bark, which will be used to extract oil from. You have likely already experienced the pleasure an essential oil can promote.

When you get a bouquet of roses or see a gorgeous flower arrangement, what is the first thing you do? Most of you will say you stop and give the flowers a good sniff. You want to smell the aroma of the roses. When you make a mint tea or chop up peppermint for your favorite dish, you are greeted with the sweet, fragrant smell that instantly invigorates you. That is mint essence. What if you could capture that scent and have it available whenever you wanted without hunting high and low for fresh mint or fresh flowers? You can and that is why we are lucky to have essential oils available to us.

Essential oils are that fragrance you appreciate from the peppermint leaves or rose petals. When the plants are put through an extraction process, the result is a very concentrated liquid. The liquid is typically clear and is packaged and sold as an essential oil. A drop of essential oil will go a long way. Ironically, the "oil" isn't really oily at all and has more of a watery look and feel. They are referred to as oils because of the similarity in properties.

Essential oils tend to have very weak water solubility levels, meaning they don't dissolve in water. Another similar trait is the fact the oils evaporate into the air very quickly. Because of this, essential oils are often referred to as "volatile oils." Note, this does not mean they are unstable, but rather they have an affinity to evaporate rapidly.

1

It is important to clarify essential oils are not the same as oils used to make perfumes. Perfume oils are chemically produced, while essential oils are natural. Only essential oils hold any kind of therapeutic qualities.

How Oils are Made

As with any product on the market, there is a big difference in the quality of oils currently on the shelves today. It is important to point out that there is no government agency that oversees or regulates the production of essential oils. Therefore, you should only buy from trusted companies. The way an essential oil is produced does matter.

Distilling is the most common method of obtaining a plant's essence. However, it is a process that cannot be rushed. It is a slow, tedious process and as you can imagine, anything that requires a great deal of time to produce is going to be expensive. The first time you go shopping for essential oils, you need to be prepared. The oils are typically sold in small 1-ounce bottles and can cost anywhere from $5 to $20 a vial.

Almost all plants must be distilled in order to extract the oils, but there are a handful that need to be squeezed in a process referred to as cold pressing. Most citrus oils will need to be extracted with this process. It takes a lot of plants, root, bark or whatever part of the plant that is being used to make one small vial. Again, you can see why the costs tend to be high.

To distill a plant, it is crucial to the quality of the oil that only the best, healthiest plants are used. Plants should be free of disease and parasites in order to guarantee the best quality. Ideally, freshly cut organic plants should be used. All of these factors contribute to the total cost of the oil.

Steam is typically the method of choice to distill plants. Water distillation is an option, but the heat needed to extract the oil can create subpar results. If water distillation is used, ideally the process should be done with a vacuum that will allow the water to boil at a temperature less than 100 degrees Fahrenheit. This will prevent the beneficial material in the plant from being broken down or destroyed.

As the plant material is heated, the essence evaporates into steam before cooling down and turning into the oils you buy in the store today.

Making Your Own Oils

For those of you who are very hands on and like to do things yourself, you can certainly make your own essential oils. However, it is a difficult process and will require a lot of trial and error. The potency of homemade oils is often not as strong as those you would buy from a manufacturer. In the long run, it is often cheaper and easier to buy the oils than to buy the equipment needed and go through the hassle of actually making the oils. However, with that said, there are some oils that are fairly quick and simple to make if you really want to give it a try.

For the person who is interested in creating their own essential oils, let's start by saying citrus oils are the easiest. Dried orange and lemon rinds can be soaked in vodka for a few days before being strained through a coffee filter or cheesecloth. Let the liquid sit in a jar for a few more days so the alcohol can evaporate. The liquid left in the jar will be your essential oil.

Another option you have if you are not quite ready to make or buy a distiller is to use an old crockpot. It would be a good idea to have a crockpot dedicated to your essential oil making. Essential oils can be toxic, so you wouldn't want to cook a pot roast in a pot that had cooked up a toxic, potentially lethal oil. It is always better to be safe, than sorry.

Place the plant material into a crockpot with enough distilled water to cover the plants. A quick tip about using your own plant material, you will want to "bruise" the plants before you begin processing them. You can compare it to using a meat tenderizer on a steak. This helps them release the essence. It is also a good idea to use dry plants. Wet plants can grow mold and ruin your oil.

Put the crockpot on low and allow the mixture to slowly cook for a full 24 hours. After the 24 hours are up, turn off the crockpot, remove the lid and let the mixture sit for seven days in the crockpot. Just stick it off in a corner on the counter or somewhere it won't be in the way and won't be at risk of having stuff dropped into it.

You will see oil slowly start floating to the surface of the mixture. After seven days, run the oil mixture through cheesecloth and into a clean, sterile mason jar. Transfer the oil from the mason jar into a dark or amber-colored jar and allow the oil to sit uncovered for another week. DO NOT USE PLASTIC OR CLEAR JARS! The oil is corrosive and can eat through plastic, leaving you with a big mess! Also, light will break down the oil, which is why it needs to be placed in a dark jar.

Once the oil has finished "breathing," add a lid and store in a cool, dark place. Make sure you label your oils appropriately and include a production date. You can learn more about how to store your oils in chapter seven.

Chapter 2 - History of Essential Oils

Essential oils have experienced a boost in popularity as more people move to natural methods of healing some of their ailments. While essential oils are currently becoming a popular trend, they have been around for quite some time. In fact, the use of essential oils has been a normal practice in some cultures for many centuries.

We can trace essential oils back to at least 1500 B.C. The Bible names frankincense as one of the oils delivered to baby Jesus to celebrate his birth. Throughout the Old and New Testaments, the use of essential oils is referenced for their healing properties as well as used for cleaning.

The ancient Egyptians used oils for a variety of rituals and healing, including a key role in the embalming process. The Egyptians relied heavily on essential oils in their daily lives. The oils were regularly used in bathhouses and in the homes of the upper members of society as fragrances.

Ancient cultures knew of the disinfectant qualities of essential oils long before the need for antiseptics were ever introduced. China and India quickly implemented the use of essential oils, herbs and plants the oils were derived from into their healing methods. In the 1800s, a text was found that listed over 800 different combinations of essential oils that were used to treat various ailments. These discoveries have been passed down throughout the centuries. They have evolved as more cultures experimented with the oils and realized even more powerful properties of the natural healing aids.

An interesting part of history that you may have heard of was the devastation the Bubonic Plague caused. It was often referred to as the Black Death. It swept across Europe killing thousands of people. One particular group took advantage of the high number of deaths and subsequent burials and robbed the tombs of the deceased. Because essential oils and other herbs were regularly entombed with the dead along with jewelry and other valuables, the thieves hit pay dirt in more ways than one.

It is likely they stole the oils and other treasure to sell for a profit, but in the process they also covered themselves in the various oils. As a result, they managed to escape the Black Death because of the medicinal qualities of the oils they stole.

Throughout time, oils have played a role in various cultures. However, in the modern era they have often been branded as "snake oils" and deemed ineffective. Oddly enough, as medical research continued forward and new discoveries were being made, essential oils became less popular. Before long they were pushed out of the medical world altogether. Thousands of years of research was ignored in favor of the latest and greatest synthetic medicines and a more intimate knowledge of the human body.

It hasn't been until the last 100 years or so that essential oils have been researched and studied to prove their value. With so many side effects to Western medicines, more and more people are turning to essential oils to learn more about them and take advantage of their natural therapeutic qualities. We now find ourselves in a world where people are quickly learning our ancestors may have been on the right track, and are, therefore, going back to the basics.

In the early 1900s, a man who was not convinced by all the hype of natural medicines learned from personal experience how useful oils were for treating wounds. He was working in his lab when he burnt his hand. He reached for the first thing he could find, which happened to be lavender essential oil. He rubbed it onto the burn and realized the pain stopped and healing was much quicker than he would have anticipated. He also noted he didn't develop an infection which is so common with severe burns.

In the 1950s, Marguerite Maury took essential oils to the next level. She had a medical background and was interested in learning how to make essential oils a part of her healing. She studied old literature and managed to figure out she needed to put the oils into a carrier oil for application to the skin. She devoted her life to the art of aromatherapy. Her work tended to focus on oils keeping a person young and beautiful in spirit. Around the same time she was studying the cosmetic benefits of oils, a man named Jean Valnet was experimenting with their medicinal values. He treated soldiers in World War II with essential oils to cure conditions like gangrene and standard injuries.

In the past 30 years or so, aromatherapy and the use of essential oils continues to intrigue scientists and alchemists. It is impossible to deny thousands of years of research and application. There is clearly a value to the plants that surround us. Essential oils are still viewed as an "alternative medicine" and will likely never be prescribed by a Western educated doctor, but you can do the necessary research and discover the value of these wonderful oils. They are truly too good to ignore.

Unfortunately, there isn't a lot of money to be made off of the production of essential oils. Drug companies are not going to spend millions of dollars researching the value and effectiveness of something that grows in the wild. Something that nearly anybody can get their hands on.

Just because big pharmaceutical companies won't spend the time, energy or money researching essential oils, it doesn't mean you cannot. When you think about it, hundreds, even thousands, of years before we had antibiotics and other medicines used to treat various health problems, people still lived relatively healthy lives. They did so because they had a way to take care of their health concerns. You cannot argue with the results of time-tested therapies. Our ancestors used essential oils and we can too.

Chapter 3 - Why Use Essential Oils

It is becoming increasingly clear that not all Western medicine is entirely safe. The list of side effects that accompany some medicines is often scarier than the condition they are being used to treat. It seems a little senseless to take an over-the-counter medicine to help clear up our nasal passages that could put us at risk of a heart attack or stroke. Or equally as impractical to give our children a medicine meant to help calm them that carries the risk of giving the child a severe disability. Sometimes, it isn't worth the risk. However, please don't take this as a blatant disregard for Western medicines. Many are deemed safe and can make a person's quality of life better and help them to live longer.

You may have also heard a lot about new strains of antibiotic-resistant bacteria that are becoming increasingly common. These strains have mutated to the point that the antibiotics we have available to use today are ineffective at killing them. This is because we have used antibiotics as a crutch. Doctors prescribe antibiotics at an alarming rate, which has resulted in these deadly bacteria.

It's highly warranted to find and use alternatives to antibiotics so that when we have a serious infection, Western medicine will be effective. We owe it to our children to back off the antibiotics and rely on alternative medicines that are just as effective without all the hefty side effects and possibility of building up a tolerance to a specific cure.

Another very good reason to rely on essential oils to take care of some of your minor health problems is the issue of cost. Not discounting the huge time and cost investment in research and development, pharmaceutical companies still make billions of dollars every year off the drugs they manufacture. Some medicines cost thousands of dollars for a single dose. Insurance companies are quickly passing the burden on to subscribers and many people are being forced to choose between buying their medications or paying their other bills. If you could eliminate even one medication by substituting it with another that was just as effective, cheaper and safer, wouldn't you do it?

Because essential oils are a natural product, no one person or company can own the rights to it or patent them. This means no one company is going to get rich by owning the exclusive rights to a particular essential oil. If somebody was looking to get rich, confirming the benefits of natural cures would certainly not be a good move.

Many people are also opting to use essential oils for their daily cleaning routines as well. A little drop goes a long way and ultimately it is much cheaper than buying gallons of cleaning supplies, scented candles or medicinal lotions. How many cleaning agents carry dire warnings about mixing them with other solutions and warnings about breathing in the toxic fumes? It can be a little scary. If we could clean our toilets without worrying about taking out an eye or burning our hands with a toxic chemical, why wouldn't we?

Take a look at the cleaning aisle in your grocery store. Do you notice a common trait to them? Almost all cleaning products boast lemon-fresh scent or orange scents. And why is that? Because citrus oils are excellent cleaning agents! You don't have to have all the extra chemicals in the bottle to get a clean, bacteria-free home!

Most essential oils contain some amount of antibacterial, antifungal and antiviral properties. Nobody can dispute that fact, which is why it is peculiar we have ignored these valuable plants and their essence for so long! **Please note:** essential oils are not a cure all and should never be ingested unless you are a trained professional. Essential oils can be toxic! Do not ever use an oil unless you have tested it first. Before applying an essential oil salve or lotion on your skin, test a small area to ensure you will not have an allergic reaction. If you are allergic to a particular food, like oranges for example, you can pretty much bet you will be allergic to orange oil.

9

For this particular book, we are talking about using essential oils as disinfectants and topical applications. Aromatherapy will also be covered.

Essential Oils and Our Olfactory System

It is a fact that our sense of smell, or olfactory system, sends direct messages to our brain. Certain smells can make us feel better or worse. Smell also determines what we taste. This is why the powerful scents that are captured in various oils are so effective at influencing our moods. We don't have to actually consume a particular plant to benefit from its medicinal qualities. Simply smelling it is all that is needed.

Smells bypass the normal route to our brain and go straight to our emotions. According to Rachel Herz, author of "The Scent of Desire," [1] smell isn't like our other senses. When we see, feel or hear something, it takes us a few seconds to process it and decide how it makes us feel. Smell has a direct line to our emotions. She explains it as "an instantaneous response in the feeling it gives you, along with responses in physiology, mood and cognition." Your brain doesn't get a chance to filter the smell and determine which nerve response it will trigger.
As an example, think of when you smell bread baking. Does it make you hungry? Do you suddenly get a craving for lasagna? The yeast in the bread is triggering a memory, which triggers a response in your brain. You automatically correlate the smell of fresh bread with a delicious meal.

So, with that line of thinking, imagine how nice it would be if smelling something like peppermint, would give you a little mood boost? That is why essential oils are used in aromatherapy. Because certain smells trigger our brain to send out signals of happiness, calmness or pleasure, aromatherapy works. You can take care of a variety of different problems simply by letting your nose do the work for you.

Essential oils trigger immune responses as well, which is why they are used therapeutically. When you inhale the steam containing the vapors from camphoraceous [kam-fuh-**rey**-shuh s] essential oils (see Chapter 4), your lungs and bronchial area are given a cue to get to work and help your body fight off an infection.

The process is extremely fast. In fact, it only takes a few minutes for your body to inhale the essence of the oils and distribute it throughout your bloodstream. This is much faster than an over-the-counter medicine. As the blood moves through your system, every cell is given a little lift from the immune-boosting properties of an essential oil.

When you put an essential oil in a carrier oil, the body absorbs it through the skin. This process takes longer, but you can think of it as a slow-release method of delivery.

Essential oils are a natural way to fight infection without ever ingesting a pill or some other medicine that may cause some undesirable side effects. The method in which the body receives the immune system boost is non-invasive, quick and very effective.

Chapter 4 - Different Types of Essential Oils

Essential oils are typically divided up into seven different categories based on the aroma they put off. Every plant has a unique smell that can be combined with other essential oils to create a pleasant aroma. The aroma produced can be used therapeutically or simply as a room freshener. As you can imagine, some smells blend together better than others. You will discover that some oils fall into several categories.

Floral

Floral oils are typically derived from the flower petals of a given plant. One of the most common floral essential oils is lavender. Rose is another one you are probably familiar with. However, there are hundreds of different plants that produce a flower of some sort, like chamomile for example. Because the petals of a flower are so fragile, typical steam distillation is not an option. The excess heat can damage the petals and the essence of the flower petals would be lost. A process of dissolving the petals in hexane is used to create what is known as an 'absolute.' Floral waters are not the same as essential oils and are basically a diluted form of an essential oil. Floral oils are not quite as easy to discern as other oils because of their subtle aromas.

Citrus

Citrus oils tend to be used more for making a room smell fresh or for cleaning purposes. The airy, fresh scent of citrus oils is squeezed or cold-pressed from the rind of the fruit. Unlike some of the other essential oils that are derived from the leaves and stems of a plant, citrus oils smell exactly like what you smell when peeling an orange or squeezing a lemon. The oils have a strong smell that is easily identified.

When buying a citrus essential oil, it is important to buy from reputable makers. Because the oil is squeezed from the rind of the fruit, any debris on the outside of the rind is deposited into the oil. You want to have the purest oil possible. Citrus oils are referred to as phototoxic. When the oils are exposed to sunlight, they create a dangerous reaction that is toxic to the skin. Citrus oils are best used in diffusers and are rarely used topically or ingested.

Woody

Woody essential oils are a bit subjective and you may find them listed in the earthy category as well. The oils are extracted from various trees and shrubs hence their "woody" name. The oils from trees are typically derived from the heart of the tree or the root. Some trees, like the sandalwood, hold their essence in the roots. Although oil can be extracted from other parts of the trunk, the strongest oil is obtained through the roots. Steam distillation is the most common way to extract the oil. Some woody essential oils include; juniper, cypress, cedarwood and fir.

Earthy

Earthy scents are those that you would likely smell in a lush, green forest. Earthy essential oils are more masculine and are often used in various men's colognes and products. Earthy and woody scents will often cross over. It is really the opinion of the user. Some earthy essential oils would be patchouli, lemongrass and vetiver.

Spicy

Spicy essential oils are actually derived from ingredients we use today to flavor our foods. Cinnamon is a common spice we use in the kitchen and is a popular essential oil. Spicy oils are typically combined with another sweet-smelling oil to create a harmonious, energetic scent. Distillation is the most common ways of extracting the oils.

Camphoraceous [kam-fuh-rey-shuh s]

Camphoraceous oils are most commonly used in therapeutic settings. The strong odors tend to make your eyes water a bit when the pure form of the oil is inhaled. Peppermint and eucalyptus oils help open up the airways due to the camphor qualities.

Herbs

As you can guess, herb essential oils are often found in the spicy category as well. These oils are typically used in combination with floral and citrus scents for aromatic uses. Herbs like oregano and sage are put through the distilling process. The herb smells are subtle and can often be confused with one another.

Infused vs. Carrier Oils

Not all essential oils are the same. Many essential oils are too harsh to be placed directly on the skin. However, these same harsh oils, like peppermint for example, have therapeutic qualities when applied topically. In order to use the peppermint oil to heal muscle aches, you need to add it to a carrier oil that is safe to put on the skin.

Carrier oils are typically derived from nuts, seeds or the fatty portion of a plant. They are not distilled like essential oils. Because of the fatty nature of the carrier oils, they do not evaporate like the essential oils. They have a much lighter aroma because of this. Unlike essences from plants and flowers, the oil derived from nuts can go rancid after about six months, so it is important to check expiration dates on any carrier oil.

A few of the most common carrier oils and their typical uses are listed below:

Almond - moisturizes, protects and heals the skin

Coconut - non-greasy, moisturizing oil that will leave skin smooth

Grapeseed - very light, leaves a sheen when rubbed on the body

Jojoba - easily absorbed by the skin, non-greasy, excellent for sensitive skin

Olive - excellent moisturizer for hair, heavy oil

Rose hip - ideal facial moisturizer, reduces appearance of flaws

Sunflower - anti-inflammatory, protects and moisturizes the skin

Infused oils are carrier oils that have been infused with herbs. Many people choose to make these at home. Fresh or dried herbs are placed into a carrier oil and left over very low heat. Infused oils can be mixed with essential oils. Basically, the herbs add additional medicinal qualities to a topical salve or lotion. Before trying to create your own infused oil, it is important you have a good understanding of complimentary herbs.

Some herbs that are regularly used to infuse carrier oils are as follows:

Rosemary - antiseptic qualities make it an excellent treatment for skin irritations and rashes.

Peppermint - soothing qualities make it ideal for sore muscles and feet

Cinnamon - promotes circulation and can help tired leg muscles

Oregano - has anti-inflammatory properties that can help reduce swelling in the joints

It is best if you use dried herbs when making infused oils. This will give you a longer shelf life. You can buy dried herbs or dry your own from your garden. You will need about two ounces of an herb per two cups of oil.

Now, you are probably looking at these herbs and your stomach is telling you that they would be great over a plate of leafy greens. In this case, you can infuse olive oil with your favorite herbs, like basil, oregano, or rosemary and most certainly use it as a garnish. You will be getting the benefits of the herb while enjoying their rich flavors.

Chapter 5 - Using Essential Oils for the Body

Essential oils can be used in a variety of ways. We will explore some of the common uses for various essential oils in this chapter. You can use essential oils to treat a variety of complaints like dry skin, rashes, burns, muscle aches or simply for cosmetic purposes. There are really hundreds of different uses for essential oils.

A Note About Safety

It is absolutely crucial to follow strict safety guidelines when working with essential oils. Many oils are toxic to the skin and most should never be ingested. Only a person highly trained in the art of using essential oils as medicine can provide instructions on how to properly use the oils in that way. The majority of essential oils are deadly when ingested. Because they are so highly concentrated, it only takes a single drop to do serious damage. Never use essential oils directly on the skin. A carrier oil is a necessity, not an option. Pregnant women are also advised against using or exposing themselves to the majority of essential oils. It is imperative a professional's advice is followed. Again, as mentioned in Chapter 3, always test a small area to ensure you will not have an allergic reaction.

For the Body

Essential oils can be added to a carrier oil to make a therapeutic salve, an aromatic lotion or even a beautiful fragrance. The possibilities are truly endless. If you are interested in making your own soap, shampoo or other beauty products, essential oils are perfect for giving you a signature scent. If you have always loved the smell of lavender or rose, you can add a drop or two of oil into your homemade beauty product for a little extra something special. Because the oils are so aromatic, your favorite scent will stick with you throughout the day unlike synthetic fragrances that quickly evaporate.

Essential oils are very effective at treating a number of different ailments as well. Please note—there is no such thing as "therapeutic grade" essential oils. There is no government organization to control or mandate the industry so the label is meaningless. Don't pay more for a false statement.

The following are just some of the most common uses for key oils. There are literally hundreds of oils that can be used to cure nearly anything that ails you.

Plugged sinuses, cough and congestion - Add 5 or 6 drops of eucalyptus essential oil to a small pot of water and heat on the stove until it starts to steam. Lean over the pot of water and inhale the steam. It helps to put a towel over your head to direct the steam into your face. You can also put a few drops of oil in a warmer and allow the eucalyptus to go throughout the room. Alternatively, add a few drops to a vaporizer in the place you would normally put the Vicks® solution. Yet another option is to add a couple of drops to a handkerchief and place it under your nose and inhale. Eucalyptus is one of the fastest, safest ways to clear up congestion and can be used by anybody from infants to the elderly.

Muscle aches - Peppermint essential oil is typically the go to oil for muscle pain. It can be used in a number of different ways. Add 10 drops of the oil to a warm bath and soak for a bit. Peppermint oil can be added to a carrier oil, like almond, and rubbed on the area. You can also make a cold compress by adding a few drops of your chosen oil to a bowl of cold water. Dip a washcloth into the water and then apply to the affected area. Other essential oils that are commonly used for muscle aches include: basil, lavender, cypress, clary sage, grapefruit, chamomile and rosemary.

Toothpaste - Peppermint oil is such a versatile essential oil you will want to have a good supply on hand. It is a natural disinfectant along with a mood enhancer. If you want an inexpensive, yet effective, natural tooth cleanser and whitener, add a drop of peppermint essential oil to two tablespoons of baking soda. The baking soda whitens your teeth and the peppermint oils kills the bacteria that cause cavities. Your mouth will feel fresh, just like it would after using a brand name toothpaste infused with peppermint.

Perfume or fragrant body spray —If you have seen or used those expensive body sprays at Bath and Body Works, you have probably noticed one of the main ingredients is alcohol. Alcohol dries your skin and can cause problems for some people. You can make your own body spray tailored to your preferences that is much better for your skin. Fill a small 4-ounce spray bottle with distilled water and add about 40 drops of your favorite essential oil. Choose from lavender, rose or any other essential oil that appeals to you. You can certainly experiment by mixing several oils to create a signature fragrance. It is important you give the bottle a good shake in order to get the oil to mix with the water. You know what they say about oil and water—shake hard!

Lotion - Lavender and rose tend to be the favorite essential oils to use in lotions, but you can use whatever appeals to you. Choose a carrier oil that is thick and non-greasy. Coconut, jojoba and grapeseed are some of the most used carriers for lotions. Again, you will want to experiment a little to find a lotion that is light enough for your tastes and isn't too greasy. You will also want to experiment with the number of drops you add to the carrier lotion.

Mood Enhancer - We talked about the power of your olfactory system earlier. Certain essential oils have the power to lift your spirits and even give you a little energetic boost. Peppermint and citrus oils are perfect for this reason. However, if you need to relax a little, lavender oil is ideal. You can add a few drops of this oil to a handkerchief and pull it out from time to time at work or in the car. The effects are almost instantaneous.

Chapter 6-Essential Oils for the Home

Essential oils are regularly used in the home for cleaning, disinfecting and deodorizing. There has been an increase in popularity for homemade cleaning products. They are considered to be safer and are much more cost friendly than the thousands of products on the market today. When you make your own cleaning products, you know exactly what you are getting and don't have to worry about any allergic reactions. Plus, one or two homemade cleaning products can take the place of the 10 you probably have stored under your kitchen sink or in the laundry room. Seriously, one cleaner is usually enough.

This list is just a sample of the hundreds of different ways you can use essential oils in your home.

Room freshener - Citrus oils like orange and lemon make the ideal room fresheners. You can get the scent into the room in a couple of different ways. If you have an oil warmer add a few drops of your favorite oil and let it do the rest. You will need to add fresh drops every couple of hours on the low setting to keep the room filled with the fragrance. You can also create your own room spritzer by adding your favorite essential oil to a spray bottle filled with distilled water. You will need to add about 60 drops of oil and shake vigorously. Spray the room with a fine mist as you would with an aerosol freshener. As an extra bonus, orange oil is a natural disinfectant as are most citrus oils. When cold and flu season hits, leave the Lysol® and reach for your homemade air freshener and disinfectant.

Cleaning solution - Grab another spray bottle and fill it with water. Add a few drops of a citrus oil, like orange or lemon. Use it as a cleaning spray to wipe down kitchen countertops and the bathroom area. You really only need one cleaner and citrus oils are excellent cleansers and disinfectants.

Sachets - You can freshen your clothes by adding a few drops of essential oil to a cotton ball. Place the cotton ball in the corner of your drawers to keep them smelling fresh. Lavender is the perfect choice, but you can certainly add whatever scent speaks to you. Peppermint is a mouse deterrent. If you are having a problem with mice in your closet, try adding a few peppermint soaked cotton balls around the edge of your closet.

Carpet deodorizer - If you have pets this is an excellent tool! Grab a box of baking soda and add a few drops of lemon essential oil or another scent you appreciate and sprinkle the baking soda on an area where a pet had an accident or where they tend to lay. Let the baking soda sit for a few minutes and then vacuum. Your carpet will be left smelling fresh and clean.

Candles - If you love scented candles from some of those famous companies, you have probably realized they can get rather expensive for something you are literally going to burn. It is like burning money! You can make your own scented candles for a fraction of the price. Buy the materials necessary for making your own candles and then choose a variety of essential oils to scent the candles. You can mix and match to create the perfect scent for you. Burning candles scented with essential oils is another way for you to give your spirits a little boost. Experiment and have fun with this.

Soap - Scented soaps are very popular these days. Washing with lavender scented soap leaves your skin smelling fresh all day while giving you the benefits of the lavender oil. Making soap is another fairly easy activity. It only takes a few ingredients and is a natural product for you to use on your skin. You can make soap with floral scents for the females in your family and woody or earthy scents for the men in your family. Experiment with the various soap bases, like goat's milk, oatmeal or glycerin. Some popular oils to use in soaps include rosemary, which is an antiseptic and great for those with acne and peppermint for its soothing qualities.

Chapter 7 - Where to Buy Essential Oils

As we mentioned in the first chapter, there is a difference in the quality of essential oils on the market today. It is best to do your research before spending your money on any essential oils. Many companies will have websites established that explain their method of extraction as well as reveal where they obtain the plant material.

The climate in which the plants are grown is crucial to the quality of the oil. Ideally, you want to buy from a company that only uses the highest quality of plant material in order to have the best concentration levels. Companies that uphold quality control standards are more likely to sell the best essential oils. Do not be fooled by high prices and assume the more expensive a company's prices, the better their oils. Do some research and draw your own conclusions.

It is also important to note that oils that are mass produced will not yield the strongest results. The extraction process takes a great deal of care and any deviation can cause weak oils. The following list includes some key things you should look for when buying an essential oil.

- A label indicating the company uses 3rd party testing to determine the quality of their product.
- Oil should be clear except for a couple of citrus oils.
- Region plants were grown is listed on the label or packaging.
- Vendor is willing to answer specific questions about the extraction process.
- Organic oils are superior to non-organic. If an oil is organic, it should be specified on the label.

Essential oils are typically sold at specialty stores and are not commonly found in the standard department stores or pharmacies. You can also buy the oils online, which gives you the opportunity to look for the best prices as well as have a wider selection of oils to choose from. Ideally, you want to buy from smaller companies. This ensures you are getting a product that is not being produced en masse and is likely going to be of a higher quality. With that said, the smaller companies do tend to charge a bit more because of the lower yields.

Some companies that sell essential oils are as follows:

http://www.bulkapothecary.com/categories/aromatherapy-essential-oils.html?gclid=CKbUyP6_nL4CFceCfgodzgUAAg

https://www.mountainroseherbs.com/catalog/aromatherapy

http://www.organicinfusionswholesale.com/organic-essential-oils.html?gclid=CMj4hbjAnL4CFQeVfgodKb8ApQ

http://www.nowfoods.com/Products/Products-by-Category/Aromatherapy/

You can also find some pretty good deals on Amazon and eBay. Just make sure you only buy from reputable sellers. You can test just how pure an oil is from a seller. Put a drop of oil on a piece of construction paper. If the oil evaporates quickly and doesn't leave a ring where it was dropped, it is fairly pure. This would indicate a high quality oil and you can add that seller to your favorite list. Oils that leave a mark on the paper have had some kind of filler added.

Storing Oils

It is important you store your oils correctly in order to preserve their therapeutic qualities. The following tips will ensure you are getting the most out of your oils and the money you spent buying them. When stored properly, you can expect to keep your oils for up to 5 years.

* Room temperature will suffice, but you must be careful the oils don't get too hot. It would be best if you avoided storing the oils in a cupboard next to the stove or directly above a heat source.

* You will also want to choose a place that will not expose the oils to direct sunlight. This can heat the oils and cause them to deteriorate. Always store your oils with the lids on. This will prevent moisture in the air from getting into the oil as well as prevent the oil from evaporating.

* Most essential oils are sold in dark brown or amber-colored bottles. This helps prevent the oils from breaking down from exposure to the light. Never store your oils in plastic. Essential oils are very powerful and can actually erode plastic.

* You have probably also noticed essential oils are sold in very small amounts. If you have purchased a larger bottle of oil and notice it is less than half-full, it is a good idea to transfer the remaining contents into a smaller bottle. This will help cut down on air oxidization.

* If you buy additional oils to stock, make sure you rotate the old ones to the front and place the new ones behind your existing supply. It would be a shame to waste oils due to a lack of proper rotation. An easy way to remember is the phrase, "First In, First Out."

10 Essential Oils You Must Have

Now that you are ready to start using essential oils, you have probably realized there are quite a few to choose from. It can be overwhelming at first when you browse through an online store or visit your local supply store. Relax and take a deep breath, you don't have to buy every essential oil available. You wouldn't want to do that, because not all oils will appeal to you. Start small and add oils as you get the hang of how to use them.

These are 10 oils you will want to have in your cupboard:

Peppermint

Eucalyptus

Orange

Lavender

Tea Tree

Lemon

Oregano

Chamomile

Frankincense

Grapefruit

These 10 oils can be used for hundreds of different things for the home and for your body. Orange and lemon are often interchangeable and it will depend a great deal on your personal preference. We talked about the different categories of essential oils. These oils are often interchangeable depending on what you have on hand and personal preference.

Conclusion

Thank you again for purchasing this book! I hope the information contained herein was useful in helping you discover the many benefits of using essential oils. As you now know, Essential Oils provide us with a natural way to enhance our lives and heal our ailments. There are literally hundreds of ways these oils can be used for the body and around the home. Thousands of years of humans successfully using these precious liquids has proven their worth.

I trust you are now ready to confidently begin using essentials oils following the numerous helpful tips and guidance included in this book. You'll no doubt benefit from incorporating essential oils in your daily life.

Also, if you enjoyed this book, please take the time to share your thoughts and post a review on Amazon. I would greatly appreciate it!

Finally, get your copy of my follow-up book, **Essential Oils and Aromatherapy Recipes: Natural Health and Beauty Solutions Using Essential Oils and Aromatherapy for Stress Reduction, Pain Relief, Skin Care, and Beauty** that has over 177 recipes for using Essential Oils to enhance your health and beauty.

PS: You didn't forget to get your FREE GIFT did you? Here's the link again just in case:

"28 Aromatherapy Recipes for Essential Oils"

This gift is the perfect complement to this book so just head over to this web address to get access.

http://www.softpresspublishing.com/aromatherapy

References

http://www.naha.org/explore-aromatherapy/about-aromatherapy/how-are-essential-oils-extracted/

http://naturalfamilytoday.com/health/what-are-essential-oils/

http://www.essentialoils.co.za/extraction-methods.htm

http://www.thehippyhomemaker.com/which-essential-oil-companies-should-you-buy-from-my-surprising-findings-on-my-quest-to-find-the-best/

http://mountainroseblog.com/essential-oil-storage-tips/

http://www.everythingessential.me/AboutOils/History.html

http://www.dummies.com/how-to/content/understanding-essential-oils.html

http://www.thesoslab.com/facts-part-1.asp

http://www.aromaweb.com/essentialoils/citrusessentialoils.asp

http://www.essentialoils.co.za/aroma-families.htm

http://www.snowlotus.org/woody-essential-oils.aspx

http://www.edenbotanicals.com/sandalwood-essential-oil.html

http://www.aromaweb.com/articles/whatcarr.asp

http://www.nourishingtreasures.com/index.php/2013/03/08/essential-oils-101-using-essential-oils-for-muscle-related-pain-relief/

http://www.edensgarden.com/101-ways-to-use/

http://www.quinessence.com/history_of_aromatherapy2.htm

http://www.essential-oil-mama.com/make-your-own-essential-oil.html

http://blahblahmagazine.com.au/orange-essential-oil/

http://www.crunchybetty.com/21-things-you-should-know-about-essential-oils

http://www.offthegridnews.com/2012/04/09/how-to-make-your-own-essential-oils-and-perfumes/

http://www.everythingessential.me/Hints/CarrierOils.html

http://pumpsandiron.com/2014/01/13/why-rosehip-seed-oil-is-my-skincare-superstar-health-benefits-and-uses/

http://birchhillhappenings.com/v1522012immune.htm

[1]http://www.energytimes.com/pages/departments/1105/holistic1105.html

9741904R00022

Printed in Great Britain
by Amazon.co.uk, Ltd.,
Marston Gate.